APPLE CIDER VINEGAR
HEALTH SYSTEM

Learn These Powerful Health Qualities . . . for a Supple, Painfree, Tireless, Ageless Body!

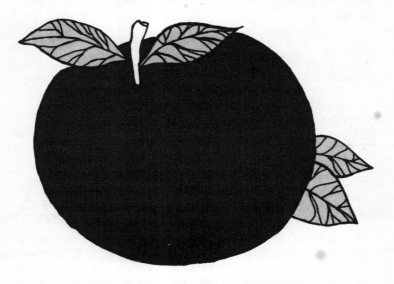

SPECIAL SUPPLEMENT!
The Bragg Blueprint for Physical, Mental and Spiritual Improvement

<u>JOIN</u> 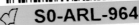 S0-ARL-964

The Bragg Crusades for a 100% Healthy, Better World for All!

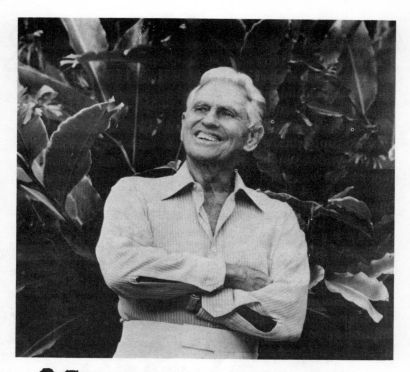

PAUL C. BRAGG, N.D., Ph.D.

Life Extension Specialist, World Health Crusader, Pioneer Nutritionist, one of the world's foremost authorities on scientific nutrition and physical fitness, at his home in Hawaii.

JOIN THE FUN AT THE "LONGER LIFE, HEALTH AND HAPPINESS CLUB" WHEN YOU VISIT HAWAII

Be sure to visit the "Longer Life, Health and Happiness Club" at Fort DeRussy, right at Waikiki Beach, Honolulu, Hawaii. Membership is free and open to everyone who wishes to attend any morning Monday through Saturday from 9:00 to 10:30 a.m. for deep breathing, exercising, meditation, group singing and mini-health lectures on how to live a long, healthy life! The group averages 75 to 100 per day. When Paul and Patricia Bragg are away lecturing, they have their leaders carry on until their return. Thousands have visited the club from around the world and then they carry the message of health and happiness to their friends and relatives back home. Paul and Patricia extend an invitation to you and your friends to join the club for health and happiness fellowship with them . . . when you visit Hawaii!

APPLE CIDER VINEGAR
HEALTH SYSTEM

SPECIAL SUPPLEMENT!
The Bragg Blueprint for Physical,
Mental and Spiritual Improvement

By
PAUL C. BRAGG, N.D., Ph.D.
LIFE EXTENSION SPECIALIST
and
PATRICIA BRAGG, N.D., Ph.D.
LIFE EXTENSION NUTRITIONIST

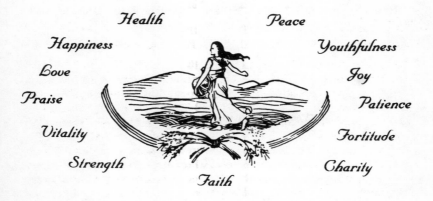

Health   *Peace*

Happiness   *Youthfulness*

Love   *Joy*

Praise   *Patience*

Vitality   *Fortitude*

Strength   *Charity*

Faith

HEALTH SCIENCE
Box 7, Santa Barbara, California 93102 U.S.A.

APPLE CIDER VINEGAR
HEALTH SYSTEM

SPECIAL SUPPLEMENT!
The Bragg Blueprint for Physical, Mental and Spiritual Improvement

By
PAUL C. BRAGG, N.D., Ph.D.
LIFE EXTENSION SPECIALIST
and
PATRICIA BRAGG, N.D., Ph.D.
LIFE EXTENSION NUTRITIONIST

Copyright © by Health Science. ~ All rights reserved under the International Copyright Union. Printed in the United States of America. No portion of this book may be reproduced or used in any manner without the written permission of the publisher, except by a reviewer who wishes to use brief quotations in a review for a magazine, newspaper, or radio or television program. For information address Health Science, Box 7, Santa Barbara, California, 93102, USA.

— REVISED —

Copyright © Health Science
Thirty-sixth printing MCMLXXXVII

ISBN: 0-87790-039-6

Health Science - Box 7, Santa Barbara, CA 93102

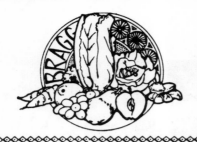

CONTENTS

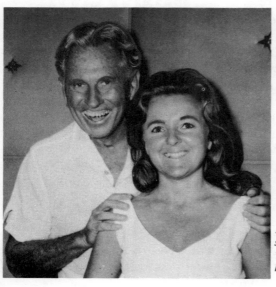

LIFE'S GREATEST TREASURE IS RADIANT HEALTH

Paul C. Bragg and daughter Patricia say, "There is no substitute for Health. Those who possess it are richer than kings."

KEEP YOUNG BIOLOGICALLY WITH EXERCISE AND GOOD NUTRITION

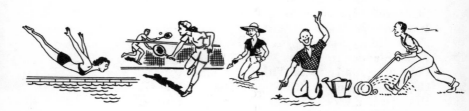

You can always remember that you have the following good reason for sticking to your health program:

- The ironclad laws of Nature.
- Your common sense which tells you that you are doing right.
- Your aim to make your health better and your life longer.
- Your resolve to prevent illness so that you may enjoy life.
- By making an art of life, you will be young at any age.
- You will retain your faculties and be hale, hearty, active and useful far beyond the ordinary length of days, and you will also possess superior mental and physical powers.

HOW TO USE THE POWERFUL HEALTH QUALITIES OF PURE NATURAL APPLE CIDER VINEGAR

Pure natural undistilled cider vinegar can really be called one of Nature's most perfect foods*

Pure natural cider vinegar must be made from fresh crushed apples and allowed to ripen or mature. It is best matured in wooden barrels, as the woods seems to "boost" the natural fermentation. Natural cider vinegar should be a dark colour and if held to the light one should see a formation of a cob-web like substance which is called the "mother." The more natural the cider vinegar, the more "mother" shows in the bottle. When you smell natural cider vinegar there should be a heavy pungent odor. I have smelt natural vinegar so natural and ripened it puckered your mouth.

WHY HAS PURE, NATURAL, FULLY AGED CIDER VINEGAR ALMOST DISAPPEARED FROM THE GROCER'S SHELVES?

The blame for the disappearance of pure natural cider vinegar from the general grocery market lies on the shoulders of the general public as well as the producers of vinegar.

Most people buy food with their eyes and not their knowledge of nutrition. The vinegar producers failed to enlighten the general public on what powerful health qualities were locked within natural cider vinegar. Most of them had not the *slightest* knowledge of the health value of cider vinegar. They produced vinegar because the public demanded it. It was simply filling supply and demand.

*Available at most Health Food Stores.

You cannot completely blame the producers of vinegar. They are not nutritionists, they are not bio-chemists. They give the public what they want.

Most people when purchasing vinegar purchase it for flavoring their foods. Some purchase it like many women to rinse their hair after shampooing as it makes the hair soft and easy to manage. Some purchase it to put in water to wash windows. There are many household uses for vinegar. So, the general public had no conception of the health value of vinegar. The producers had not the slightest idea that vinegar was a powerful and wonder-working health food. Both the general public and the producers of vinegar were in total darkness as to the powerful Health Qualities of pure, natural, fully ripened cider vinegar. Ignorance is bliss. When the general public saw pure natural cider vinegar with the dark color and the dark "mother" floating in it, it did not have eye appeal. The "mother" in the dark natural cider vinegar looked unappetizing. The general public has been educated and brain washed to want everything they purchase to have eye appeal.

To meet this demand that vinegar be bright colored and free from the dark "mother" they distilled the vinegar. In distilling, the vinegar is turned to steam by heating, therefore destroying the powerful enzymes and distilling out the powerful life giving minerals such as potassium, phosphorus, chlorine, natural organic sodium, magnesium, sulphur, iron, copper, natural organic fluorine, silicon and many other powerful trace minerals.

But the distilling also destroyed the powerful natural malic acid which is so very important in fighting body toxins.

You can plainly see that when the general public with their obsession for "eye appeal foods" and the producers of cider vinegar agreed to sell their product for a profit, it sounded the death warrant for pure natural fully ripened cider vinegar.

The public got just what they wanted, beautiful but dead vinegar. Now that natural cider vinegar was almost completely off the market other strange vinegars started to

2

appear on the market. The first being a vinegar called malt vinegar. Malt vinegar is a refined, processed vinegar. It has none of the qualities of natural vinegar. It tasted like vinegar . . . it was pure and white looking and the general public purchased it.

Then came the real tragedy—some food chemist produced an imitation vinegar from coal tar. It looked white and pure and it tasted like vinegar, now it has the biggest sale of all vinegars in the groceries. It was cheaper than distilled vinegar or malt vinegar. Today most people purchase this synthetic vinegar. There is nothing to say about this vinegar except that it is pretty to look at and tastes like vinegar, but has absolutely no health value.

So, here we have three types of vinegar on the general market. None of them has the nutritional and health values of pure, natural, fully ripened cider vinegar.

Millions of people the world over never get the health qualities of good, wholesome, natural cider vinegar.

MORE AND MORE PEOPLE SUFFER FROM MALNUTRITION

"Mal" means bad. As a consequence of not getting natural, healthful, balanced diets, millions the world over suffer from many forms of sub-clinical malnutrition. Sub-clinical malnutrition means that many people, due to mineral and vitamin deficiencies, feel half-sick most of the time. They lack vim, vigor and the "go power" to carry on the ordinary duties of life without feeling tired out most of the time.

They do not get in their vinegar or their daily foods the proper number of minerals and vitamins their bodies require. They lack vital power. They drag themselves through the day feeling exhausted most of the time. That is the reason they turn to stimulants such as tea, coffee, alcohol, cola drinks and cigarettes, and many of them, to drugs that "pep" them up for a while. After the effects of these stimulants wear off, they feel terrible. They just exist, they do not live.

3

You see these miserable people about you every day of your life. They are "washed-out" and prematurely old. They lack skin tone and muscle tone. They have black circles and big puffs under their eyes. The eyes have lost the sparkle of youthfulness. They have the "dead fish eyed look." Malnourished people are lifeless and everything they do requires a tremendous effort. They are not really living. Malnourished people are not happy people. Many of them suffer from depression and mental fatigue.

THE APPLE IS A POWERFUL FOOD NUTRITIONALLY

"An apple a day keeps the doctor away" is a familiar trite saying, but it carries truth and good common sense, because the apple is one of God's great and wonderful foods.

As stated it has one of the richest sources of potassium, and potassium is to the soft tissues of the body what calcium is to the bones and harder tissues of the body. It is the mineral of youthfulness. Potassium is the "artery softener," it keeps the arteries of the body flexible and resilient. It is a fighter of dangerous bacteria and viruses. Yes, when you say "An apple a day keeps the doctor away" you are talking good down-to-earth vital nutrition.

The apple has stood the test of time . . . it is one of the oldest fruits that man consumes.

It was in the garden of Eden that the apple played such a vital part in the destiny of man.

Man has been an apple eater for thousands of years. Apple eaters have a certain healthfulness that the non-apple eater never ever achieves.

THE APPLE – A RICH SOURCE OF POTASSIUM

While the apple is a delicious fruit and most people enjoy eating apples . . . I look on the apple as something more than something good to eat.

To me as a bio-chemist it is the key mineral in the constellation of minerals. It is so important to life of every living thing that without it there would be no life.

4

Most humans are deficient in potassium and it reflects in their cell tissue. Look about you . . . how many people do you see that have a live looking skin? Most people living in civilization and eating the foods of civilization have the potassium deficiency look. The skin and muscle tone is bad. The flesh does not cling firm on the boney framework of the body. Lines and wrinkles fill the face and neck. Notice the heavy flabby skin that hangs over the eyes of most people. The longer the potassium deficiency continues the prolapsing of the skin above the eye progresses, and soon people are looking out of little slits instead of wide-open eyes. Of course, the average person blames this on the fact that he has been adding more birthdays to his life. Most people attribute these physical changes in the skin and muscle tone to their advancing age.

You must have potassium to build youthful and ageless tissue. If you do not get your required amount of potassium daily, you acquire the "old age look." This is premature ageing due to a deficiency of potassium.

It is the same in the garden. Potassium is necessary to the production of the substances which give rigidity to plant stems and increase their resistance to the many diseases which attack plants.

Potassium is the power which changes seed into flower by progessive development.

If the plants are deficient in potassium, the plant stops its evolution at some intermediate stage. The first tell-tale sign of extreme potassium deficiency in a plant is cessation of growth for no discernible external reason. If the potassium deficiency is not corrected at once, the plant slowly starts to wither, turns yellows and dies. The same with an animal and a human body; when there is a deficiency in potassium there is a slow degeneration of body cells.

Many people go throughout life committing partial suicide — destroying their health, youth, beauty, talents, energies, creative qualities. Indeed, to learn how to be good to oneself is often more difficult than to learn how to be good to others.

When pure rules of business and conduct are observed, then there is true religion. Walk in the path of duty, do good to your brethren, and work no evil towards them.

INCREASING POOR HEALTH AND DISEASE, DUE TO MAN'S TAMPERING WITH OUR FOODS AND PROCESSING OUT THE VITAL POTASSIUM

Robbed Grains: The miller refines and processes our grains to get white flour which will keep for years. No vermin will eat it because it has been robbed of its potassium.

Amazing Potassium Loss In Making White Flour: The miller in milling the wheat refines out 25 important food elements, amino acids, vitamin E, bran, the rich B-complex vitamins, and entirely refines out the potassium.

Cows fed refined (degermed and *the potassium milled out*) grain died of heart failure.

The more we refine the potassium out of our foods, the sicker we get: Time and energy wasted on more sickness. There are too many social-minded people spending too much time and too much energy planning how to get more care for more sickness. All this energy should be directed into teaching our people the importance of a good diet, and to see that the eating habits are changed to conform to what we already know about nutrition.

People should be taught what the minerals mean to one's health. They should be taught that to be well they must get their daily supply of Potassium.

Disgraceful Sickness and Death Rates

Better medical facilities and wider distribution of physicians and dentists will never overcome the fundamental difficulties or make any appreciable dent in our disgraceful sickness and death rates . . . not disgraceful as compared with any other larger nation, for it is one of the lowest . . . disgraceful because it can be prevented. Teach the children in the schools how important the minerals are to their health and well-being . . . tell them how important it is to have potassium in the body every day.

PREVENTION THROUGH VITAL FOODS

It is, therefore, the prevention of sickness, largely through getting the correct nourishment in the body . . . especially the potassium.

BAD NUTRITION IS THE REASON PEOPLE ARE NOT WELL

People do not die of infectious conditions as such, but really from malnutrition that allows the germs to gain a foothold. In the non-infectious, fatal conditions or degenerative conditions, bad nutrition is the contributing cause in every instance.

When the body has its full quota of minerals including the precious potassium it is impossible for a germ to get a foothold in a healthy and powerful blood stream.

THE BODY HAS A SEED OF ETERNAL LIFE

Outside of fatal accidents there is no reason man should die. It has been definitely proven by some of the greatest scientific minds in the world, that there are no special diseases of old age. Because a person lives 60, 70, 80, or 90 years, there is no reason why he should die. Age is not toxic.

People die of some fatal condition that they have built in their bodies by not knowing the natural laws that govern the physical body.

The two great enemies of life are toxic poisons and nutritional deficiencies. Every 90 days a new blood stream is built in the body by the food you eat, the liquid you drink and the air you breathe. From the blood stream the body cells are made and nourished.

Every eleven months we have a new set of billions of body cells, and every 7 years we have an entirely new set of bones and hard tissues.

There is nothing to get old.

THE GREAT CARREL EXPERIMENT

In 1912 in New York City, Dr. Alexis Carrel, in his great experiment, *kept the cells of an embryo* chicken heart alive and in health for over 30 years by complete nutrition and complete elimination. The normal life-span of a chicken is 7½ to 8 years.

Cider vinegar was given the chicken embryo every day for its full daily quota of potassium.

Dr. Carrel definitely proved to the entire world that the body has a seed of eternal life. Dr. Carrel could have continued this experiment indefinitely.

It proved how important cider vinegar is to life and health.

The results of this experiment reveal the key to total health and longevity. Men of science know no reason why these same principles might not apply to human beings.

STUNTED GROWTH DUE TO POTASSIUM DEFICIENCY

I have made 13 scientific nutritional expeditions over the primitive world studying the growth of various races of people. I find where the top-soil is deficient in potassium the people living off the vegetation of the potassium deficient soil are stunted in growth.

The pygmies of Africa are stunted and short-lived people. The same with the Eskimos of the far Arctic . . . they just do not get in their daily diet the required amount of potassium . . . therefore they are stunted and short lived.

MENTALLY RETARDED CHILDREN AND ADULTS SUFFER FROM POTASSIUM DEFICIENCY

I have closely studied the relationship between mentally retarded children and adults and potassium deficiency.

Several years ago I brought 3 mentally retarded children in my home for study and observation. Each morning I gave the children a glass of water with two teaspoonsful of cider vinegar and a heaped teaspoon of honey. (Honey is a rich source of Potassium.) I worked out a carefully planned scientific diet that gave the children large amounts of Potassium. In three weeks these children became alert mentally, and after keeping them in my home one year they were able to join school again with children of their own age.

At another time I brought 4 mentally retarded adults in my home and by giving them the cider vinegar routine was able in less than one year make them self-supporting people.

They are now attending night school and are rapidly building a high I.Q.

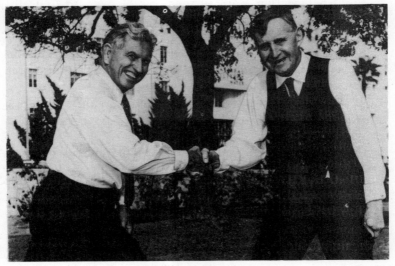

Birthdays Don't Count

Paul C. Bragg Indian wrist-wrestles with Roy White (108 years young), one of his long-time friends who lives according to Bragg's Health Principles.

Life cannot be maintained unless life be taken in, and this is best done by making at least 60 percent of your diet raw and cooked vegetables, with a plentiful supply of fresh juicy fruits. —Patricia Bragg

---

Jesus said: "Thy faith hath made thee whole, and go and sin no more." and that means your dietetic sins. He himself, through fasting and prayer, was able to heal the sick and cure all manner of diseases.

SENILITY AND
POTASSIUM DEFICIENCY

Today the world over there are hundreds of thousands of prematurely old, senile people. They are the forgotten people. Many of these people do not know their own name nor can they recognize their family or closest old friends.

They are just living human vegetables.

To me old senile people are the most pitiful people on earth. They just exist.

Some of them have so degenerated that it is hopeless to try and salvage them.

But I believe that many of them can be restored to useful lives again if the toxic poison can be flushed from their bodies and the grave deficiencies can be corrected.

Several years ago I selected six of these senile people who I believed could be salvaged. They were given their cider vinegar daily and fed foods rich in potassium.

Out of the six I was able to salvage four of them. All four left the old-age institution they had been confined in and became self-sufficient.

One of the men made a remarkable recovery . . . he actually went back to contracting and building again . . . and he was 83 years of age.

Most of these senile people were suffering from clogged arteries. Potassium is to the soft tissues of the body what calcium is to the hard structures of the body. The potassium went into those clogged and caked arteries and cleaned out the rust and dirt. No one can think normally if the arteries are heavily clogged with rust and toxic poison.

Potassium might be called the great detergent of the arteries. There is little doubt that potassium slows up the hardening and the clogging processes that menace the whole important blood vessel system. Because the potassium present in pure, natural, ripened cider vinegar makes the flesh of the dairy cow or bull tender when it is slaughtered for meat, there is very little doubt that one of the functions of potassium is to keep the tissues soft and pliable.

10

HERE ARE SOME OF THE TELL-TALE SIGNS
OF POTASSIUM DEFICIENCY

● There are aches and pains in the lower back . . . both in the bones and the muscles especially in the lower back.

● There are shooting pains when a person starts to straighten up after leaning over.

● There is dizziness when you straighten up after leaning over.

● A dull morning headache upon arising.

● The body feels heavy and it is an effort to move rapidly.

● The hair is dull and faded looking, it lacks lustre and sheen, the scalp is itchy, there is dandruff and premature balding.

● The hair is unmanageable and mats up and often looks like straw. Sometimes it is extremely dry, and another time it feels like it is oil soaked.

● The eyes itch and feel sore at times, sometimes the eye lids are granulated and white matter runs from the eyes. At other times the eyes are heavily blood-shot and watery.

● The eyes tire easily and will not focus as they should.

● There is an extreme loss of mental alertness, making decisions hard to make. The memory seems to fail, making you forget names and places that should be at the tip of your tongue. You become very forgetful. You tire physically and mentally with the slightest effort.

● You become impatient and sometimes very irritable to your loved ones.

● You feel nervous and have periods of depression and mental fog. You just cannot get things done, due to mental and muscle fatigue. The slightest effort sometimes leaves you shaking and trembling.

● At times the hands and the feet get cold, even in warm weather. There are many other symptoms of potassium deficiency.

PURE NATURAL CIDER VINEGAR
IS ONE OF THE GREATEST SOURCES OF POTASSIUM

Long years of research have proved to me that natural apple cider vinegar is a potent source of potassium.

When I was a small boy I was reared on a large farm. On this farm we grew many varieties of apples. I was a great apple eater. I enjoyed robust health. My father each year made pure apple cider vinegar and stored it in wooden barrels. On our table we used this pure apple cider vinegar and the whole family (I am the oldest of 16 children) liked vinegar.

My father was a splendid farmer and many times I would watch him add cider vinegar to the feed of ailing cattle. It acted like magic. The vinegar seemed to possess some magic ingredient that could help restore health to the cattle again.

The nearest doctor was 32 miles from our home. If a doctor was needed the doctor had to drive by horse and buggy over miles of rough rugged poor roads.

So, at our home we developed a sort of home folk medicine and vinegar played an important role.

I well remember when my father put in long hours at farm work during the harvest period. He was up long before day break and would not retire until late at night.

I would watch him come into our kitchen, put a heaping teaspons of honey in a glass, then add 2 teaspoons of pure apple cider vinegar and then fill the glass with water.

I would say "Father, why do you drink honey, vinegar and water?" And father would reply, "Son, farm work is hard work, it produces chronic fatigue in the body. Whatever is in this mixture relieves me of that chronic fatigue."

Yes, father was correct. There was an ingredient in that drink that renewed his vitality and relieved him of chronic fatigue, and that ingredient is potassium.

Most people today when they work hard turn to all kinds of dangerous stimulants to relieve their chronic fatigue. Alcohol, tobacco, coffee, tea, cola drinks and even dangerous drugs.

My father's good advice fell on youthful ears. It was some years later that I realized that my father was a smart man in using honey and cider vinegar to combat chronic fatigue.

At 12 I was sent from my healthy and rugged farm life to a large military academy and the food of that institution was where my health was broken. The refined and processed food broke me down and made me a victim of TB.

At no time did I see pure natural apple cider vinegar or honey at the table of our military academy.

It was not until I met the great Doctor Rollier at the sanitarium in Switzerland that I came in contact with the miracle of cider vinegar and honey, both of which are so rich in essential potassium.

When I arrived at the sanitarium I was given each morning the same drink my father took at the farm for chronic fatigue.

Potassium is a hard fighter against germs, and I owe much of my recovery to apple cider vinegar and honey.

Dr. Rollier urged us to put cider vinegar on our raw salads. He urged us to use an abundance of honey each day. He was a wise doctor. He knew how valuable potassium was to the body chemistry.

Along with a perfectly balanced natural diet, correct breathing, and Alpine sunshine I was a 100% cured case of TB in less than two years.

Since that day so many years ago, I have been an ardent user of cider vinegar and honey and in my health teachings and writings have advocated the use of these splendid sources of potassium.

CIDER VINEGAR FOR OVERWEIGHT

I want it understood that cider vinegar will not reduce a person who does not control the intake of food, but when combined with a diet of from 1200 to 1500 calories a day it will help and assist in the reduction of excess weight. The vinegar and honey cocktail should be taken 3 times daily. It consists of ½ teaspoon of honey, 2 teaspoons of cider vinegar in a glass of water.

Along with this cocktail there must be exercise and a reducing diet. That means that all breads, cereals and dairy products are eliminated from the diet. The diet should consist of fruit, raw salads, cooked 5 per cent vegetables such as string beans, spinach or any other greens, cooked celery, cooked squash, lean meat and fish.

COMBATING UNDERWEIGHT WITH
CIDER VINEGAR & HONEY

Cider vinegar is proving to be one of the greatest aids to health, known to science, it is an entirely natural substance, produced by powerful enzymes (Life Chemicals).

The underweight person is deficient in these powerful enzymes and therefore cannot use or burn up the food that is put into the body. No matter how much fatty food, protein or any other kind of food is put into the body it is not used by the body.

As long as there is a deficiency of enzymes there is going to be underweight. The underweight person should use the following cocktail on arising: 2 teaspoons of cider vinegar, 1 heaping teaspoon of honey, to one glass of water.

The underweight person should add one drop of Lugols solution to the above mixture. Lugols will add Iodine to the body which is very important in adjusting body weight.

RIDDING THE BODY OF DANGEROUS
TOXIC WASTES
CELL PURIFYING

Toxic poisons are the cause of most troubles in the human body. Most people do not have the *vital force* to supply the eliminative organs with the strength to move the normal waste from the body. Without this energy the wastes

14

are not flushed from the body. There they remain and lodge in the joints and organs of the body. We have a name for each symptom that gives us pain and trouble. Certain toxic wastes that are harmful to the whole body are rendered harmless by a substance in cider vinegar.

Scientists call this protective action *"Acetolysis."*

Waste products by this process are broken down, then made harmless. When you feel badly and do not seem to have the *"Go Power"* to do the things in life that are necessary, it is then time to flush out some of the toxic wastes that the organs of elimination cannot seem to handle.

Remember the organs of elimination are the bowel, the lungs, the skin and the kidneys. They are your faithful servants. They work hard 24 hours daily flushing out toxic wastes. Many times these eliminative organs must have help and that is when cider vinegar comes to their aid.

DIRECTIONS FOR BODY PURIFICATION WITH CIDER VINEGAR

To six ounces of tomato juice add 2 teaspoons of natural cider vinegar. Drink between meals, once or twice daily.

RELIEVING HEADACHES WITH CIDER VINEGAR

People blame their headaches on many different organs of the body. Most headaches are blamed on the eyes, the nerves, the liver, the sinuses, the stomach, the bowels and kidneys. Headaches can be put in two classifications.

One type of chronic headache can be associated with long standing disease. The headache is a messenger telling the person that deep down in their body, destruction is going on, and something should be done. In other words this is Nature's great warning signal. There may be trouble in the gall bladder, or the liver, the kidneys or in fact in any one of the important organs of the body.

The second type of headache is emotional. This is often caused by nervousness, anxiety, stress, strain, tension or any emotional upsets.

This is a world where we must be associated with other human beings. Our daily life with other humans can throw us into terrible emotional strains because they arouse in our being the emotions of fear, jealousy, envy, hate, greed, self-indulgence and self-pity. When our emotions reach a boiling point we end up with a dull, aching headache.

The worst of the headaches is the migraine where the head seems to be splitting apart.

I have found in my many years of research on all kinds of headaches that when the body triggers a headache the urine is alkaline rather than its normal acid. It means the kidneys are disturbed by the emotions. It means that the body is off-balance.

To aid the kidneys in getting the urine back to the normal reaction, the malic acid of cider vinegar is suggested as a relief from headaches.

Directions:

It is a vaporizing method.

In a small pan or basin put equal parts of cider vinegar and water; place on the stove allowing mixture to boil slowly. When the fumes begin to rise from the pan, put a towel over your head and lean the head over until the fumes are comfortably strong. Now take deep breaths of the cider and water mixture. Inhale them for at least 80 breaths.

Many suffers of chronic headaches have told me that they get blessed relief in 35 to 40 minutes, with this method.

I have had many people tell me that by this method of combating a headache they had completely discarded the use of pain killers and headache remedies.

CIDER VINEGAR FOR COMBATING WARTS, CORNS AND CALLOUSES

Soften and dissolve corns, callouses in palms and soles of feet, warts, by applying full strength cider vinegar to them.

Do this *after* soaking parts involved in very warm water for twenty minutes. After soaking in warm water, dry the parts well . . . apply full strength cider vinegar, using pieces of cotton that have been saturated with it. Leave cider vinegar on parts for ten minutes, then wash off with tepid water. Dry parts, then rub the corns and calloused areas briskly with a rough turkish towel.

Caution: *Do not* rub warts after washing off cider vinegar. Pat dry, gently. These precautions are taken to prevent spreading of warts.

FOR SUNBURN OR BURNS

Lightly pat the skin with cider vinegar to remove sting and burning. This will give you prompt relief. For allover sunburns, pour one to two cups of cider vinegar in warm bath water, then soak the body in the tub.

COMBATING SORE THROATS WITH CIDER VINEGAR

Cider vinegar is a dangerous enemy to all kinds of germs that attack the throat. To fight throat germs, fill a glass or cup ¼ full of cider vinegar, then fill the rest of the way with slightly warm water. Do not use hot water, or it will kill the enzymes. This is now ready to be used as a gargle. Three mouthfuls of the mixture is gargled each hour, and then spit out. Do not swallow the mixture, because the vinegar acts like a sponge, drawing out germs and toxins from the surrounding tissues. As the throat begins to feel better, intervals between gargling may be extended to once every hour and a half.

Along with the gargling, heat some water and add two tablespoons of cider vinegar, dip a cloth in the hot mixture and apply to the entire throat region and over this cloth wrap a hot towel. Let the skin of the throat absorb this mixture through the skin of the neck.

Even in good health, use of the cider vinegar gargle is recommended once or twice weekly to help remove the body toxins being eliminated through the throat tissues. The gargle is also helpful during fasting, when the throat may produce a dark, stringy mucus as part of the healing/detoxifying process!

CIDER VINEGAR FOR KEEPING THE SKIN HEALTHY

Vitality With the Vinegar Massage

In a small basin of warm water add one half cup of cider vinegar . . . now with both hands dip in the mixture and massage this all over the nude body . . . face, neck, chest, arms, shoulders, back, abdomen, legs and feet. Rub the mixture into the skin thoroughly. Be vigorous in your massage. The skin of the body when it is healthy has an acid reaction for it is throwing off toxic poisons through its billions of pores.

The reason this treatment is far better than using soap is because soap has an alkaline reaction on the skin and this is just what you do not want! Keep the skin in the acid reaction and have not only healthy skin but it will contribute to a healthy body. After thoroughly wetting the skin with the mixture several times . . . now rub and massage the skin until the skin is dry. Do this at least once a week but do not wash it off . . . leave it on the body. You will note as you massage the mixture in the skin that there will be a new vitality coming into your body.

I find after hard exercise, or long mental work that I get a new feeling of strength and energy after one of these vinegar massages. The next time you feel mentally or physically tired and worn-out, try this pep building routine with cider vinegar and water . . . I assure you, you will do it many, many times.

Benefits will speak for themselves!

CIDER VINEGAR FOR ITCHING SCALP, DRY HAIR, DANDRUFF AND BALDNESS

The highly acid—organic acid (Malic acid) plus the powerful enzymes (Life Chemicals) in cider vinegar kill the "bottle bacillus," a germ responsible for many scalp and hair conditions. The problems caused by bottle bacillus include itching scalp, dandruff, falling hair and baldness.

Every hair has its own "oil can." Bottle bacilli clog the openings. Scales and small dry crusts are formed. Itching and dandruff results. The oil-starved hairs either fall out or break off, causing thinning of the hair and baldness.

18

Cider vinegar not only kills bottle bacillus, but stimulates the "oil cans" to greater activity.

Directions:
Pour two tablespoons of cider vinegar in a small cup or bowl. Moisten a face cloth or cotton ball with water, then soak it in the vinegar. Part the hair in sections, and apply the cider vinegar directly to the scalp. Leave it on for at least fifteen minutes, up to two or three hours, before shampooing . . . this helps to restore the proper acid/alkaline balance to the scalp. For acute cases, this should be done daily, or before every shampoo.

For a healthy after-shampoo rinse, add a small amount of cider vinegar to the rinse water.

HOW TO HAVE A YOUNGER LOOKING SKIN IN FIVE MINUTES WITH CIDER VINEGAR

The skin, outside layer, consists of microscopically small flat scales that are constantly flaking off, thereby revealing *the new skin beneath the outer, older layer of scales.* In countless numbers of people, the old, dead, dry outer scales do not peel off promptly, leaving the old looking, dry, dull, lifeless skin for others to see. This is called "the old age look." *Use the cider vinegar "face peel" for sensational results and look younger.*
Directions:
First wash the skin in very warm water (no soap). Next apply a heavy towel soaked in warm water to skin for three minutes. Remove. Then after wringing out a soft linen towel in water (tepid), *containing three tablespoons of cider vinegar per cup of water*, apply to skin. Then cover the linen towel with heavy towel wrung out in very warm water. Keep on for 5 minutes.

Remove both towels. Rinse skin in warm water, then rub skin briskly with a damp turkish towel. This last "rub" is to remove the millions of old, dry skin scales that have been detached and loosened by the cider vinegar peel. This can be repeated weekly, with sensational results. Your skin will look fresh and youthful. The skin will shine with joyous new life. After all we are judged by our looks. We all have a certain pride to look our best and make a good personal appearance.

FOR SKIN BLEMISHES AND PIMPLES

First steam the face while standing over a pan of boiling water, using a towel draped over the head to trap the steam, to loosen all grease and dirt. Then pat apple cider vinegar on the skin with a cotton ball to remove the loosened dirt. Repeat twice, then pat on some chilled cider vinegar to close the pores and tone the skin. This steam cleansing should be done about once a week. (Another excellent skin cleanser is the pulp of the *aloe vera* cactus. Break off a rib of *aloe vera*, slit it open and rub the pulp directly on the skin.)

HOW TO STRENGTHEN THE HEART

Directions:
Take a little "nip" of cider vinegar (two or three drops) in a half glass of water, three times daily between meals. It is especially good before you take a walk, run or any exercise.

The heart is a large muscle. It uses large amounts of potassium to keep going strong hour after hour, your entire life. It is the hardest working muscle in your body. It must have a constant and continuous supply of power and energy to continue beating. Cider vinegar contains a natural chemical that combines with heart "fuel" to make the heart muscle much stronger. (It strengthens other muscles, also.)

FOR MUSCLE SORENESS AND ACHING JOINTS

To soothe tired aching muscles and joints, there is nothing like an apple cider vinegar bath combined with a self-massage. While soaking in a warm bath to which one or two cups of cider vinegar have been added, slowly massage the entire body, starting with the soles of the feet. Gently but firmly squeeze and relax each part of the foot, working slowly up the leg to the hip. Then begin again with the other foot. Continue up the torso, then the arms and neck, always rubbing towards the heart. For the face, lightly pat the skin in an upward direction—always avoid pulling the facial skin down. Finish up with a fingertip massage in circular motions over the scalp and head.

FOR NOSEBLEEDS

Soak a small piece of cotton in vinegar and pack it lightly in the nostril. Leave it in place while the vinegar helps the blood to congeal.

HOW TO IMPROVE THE DIGESTION
WITH CIDER VINEGAR

Five minutes before starting the meal, take one tablespoon of water to which has been added *two drops* of cider vinegar. Before swallowing this, hold it in the mouth for a few seconds. Holding it in the mouth as directed draws saliva, one of the most important digestive juices. Saliva starts digestion of starches, right in the mouth. Millions have poor starch digestion, causing gas, heart-burn, discomfort and bloating of the abdomen, because of weak saliva. In the stomach, *before meals,* the diluted cider vinegar draws the stomach digestive fluids to flow faster and better, resulting in improved digestion.

HOW TO FIGHT KIDNEY STONES
WITH CIDER VINEGAR

A large number of kidney stones are of a type that can be dissolved with cider vinegar.

Use cider vinegar freely on salads consisting of cabbage, carrots, celery, beet root, tomatoes, green onions, parsley, cucumbers. Eat prunes, raisins, apples, at the same meal with the cider vinegar on salad.

HOW TO FIGHT BLADDER INFECTIONS
WITH CIDER VINEGAR

A large dish of fresh raw tomatoes with a generous amount of cider vinegar and olive oil.

1 glass of pure apple juice with a teaspoon of cider vinegar. This must be sipped very slowly.

This combination should be used at least three times weekly.

COMBATING GALL STONES WITH CIDER VINEGAR

Before starting this gall bladder flush, for one week drink four 8 oz. glasses of apple juice straight, or diluted if hypoglycemic.

In an 8 ounce glass put one third pure olive oil (no other oil will give this reaction), two thirds pure apple juice and add one tablespoon of cider vinegar. You take this mixture three times the first day.

No food is eaten during this gall bladder flush.

On the second day you take it twice . . . on both days you may drink all the apple juice you desire . . . but no other liquid . . . not even water. On the morning of the third day eat a generous salad of raw cabbage, carrots, celery, beet root, tomatoes and lettuce with generous amounts of cider vinegar and olive oil. Eat a dish of steamed greens such as spinach, kale or any other cooked leafy greens.

Watch your bowel movements . . . and see what happens.

USING CIDER VINEGAR TO HELP SHRINK
THE PROSTATE GLAND

Directions:

With a fork "whip" one tablespoon of cider vinegar with two tablespoons of pure olive oil and a dash of cinnamon. Pour on sliced tomato. Use once or twice daily, at meals.

HOW TO USE CIDER VINEGAR
FOR FEMALE TROUBLES

For better health of the vagina, use cider vinegar douches.

Directions:

Three tablespoons of cider vinegar to two quarts of warm water. This is a cleansing, antiseptic and restorative douche.

If there is a discharge use once or twice daily, depending on severity of discharge, then less frequently as the discharge lessens. For good vaginal hygiene, use once a week.

To shrink, tighten and tone a flabby womb, eat salads made with lots of parsley, and celery, on which two tablespoons of cider vinegar are poured. Unsaturated oils may be added for flavor. Peanut, soya, sunflower, safflower and olive oil are unsaturated oils.

HOW TO FIGHT ARTHRITIS WITH CIDER VINEGAR

Hard stony deposits fill up and cement the joints. Other stony deposits enlarge and cripple the joints. Crippling, painful arthritis results!

Fight those stony deposits with cider vinegar.

Directions:

On arising have a six ounce glass of tomato juice to which one half teaspoonful of cider vinegar has been added. Follow this immediately by eating a whole raw apple. At each meal put one tablespoon of cider vinegar on a raw salad. Be sure to eat an apple at this meal.

COMBATING MUCUS CONDITIONS WITH CIDER VINEGAR

Many people are plagued with mucus from the sinus cavities, nose and throat. They have a post-nasal drip which is most uncomfortable. If these mucus sufferers will discontinue dairy products and eggs from the diet and use plenty of cider vinegar they will find that this mucus condition will disappear in time.

Directions:

On arising have a glass of water with a teaspoon of honey and two teaspoons of cider vinegar. Sometime during the day this same drink should be repeated. On two salads a day at least a tablespoon of cider vinegar should be combined with olive oil. Paprika is a rich source of potassium. It should be used on salads, and on cooked foods. Along with cider vinegar, apple juice and grape juice may be drunk between meals. The important thing is that they must be sipped very slowly. They are really foods and not beverages. A small amount in the mouth at a time will be better digested and used by the body chemistry.

CIDER VINEGAR AND CONSTIPATION

It is important that the bowels move freely. Out-go should equal intake. That is, you should have a bowel movement on arising and one within an hour after each meal. Cider vinegar and flaxseed tea acts as a lubricant to the bowels. Make a tea of two tablespoons of flaxseed . . . boil 2 cups of water and add two tablespoons of flaxseed. Boil for fifteen minutes. Then strain off the flaxseed . . . you will have a jelly-like substance. Drink a cup of this on an empty stomach to which you add one teaspoon of cider vinegar. Use this everyday until you get good daily bowel movements.

Warning: Cider vinegar is not a cure for any disease. Curing is an internal biological function . . . only the body cures itself. As stated, cider vinegar is proving to be one of the greatest aids to health, known to nutritional science. It is an entirely natural substance, produced by powerful enzymes (Life Chemicals). It is the richest source of potassium and this mineral is most important to the health of the body.

With the suggestions given in the book, a natural diet should be followed. At least 50% of the diet should be composed of raw fruit and vegetables and properly cooked fruits and vegetables. There should be natural proteins, starches, sugars and fats used. All refined, processed and denatured foods should be eliminated from the diet. Tea, coffee, alcohol and cola drinks should not be put in the body chemistry.

When the body is purified of the toxins and there is no more malnutrition ("mal" means bad), the body should be healthy and working normally.

The body is self-healing and self-repairing. It is our duty if we wish a vibrant glorious health to do all we can to make the body work efficiently.

24

Not only a good diet is necessary but good habits of sleeping, out-of-door physical activity, full deep breathing and a serene mind. Man cannot live by bread alone. Man must have spiritual food. Man must strive to find a perfect balance — physically, mentally and spiritually.

WHAT BECOMES OF THE ACID CRYSTALS PRECIPITATED IN THE BODY

You have often heard the expression . . . "He's old and stiff and his flesh is tough." When we think of "old" people we think of them as stiff in the moving joints of the body and that the flesh of this old body is tough.

Why do people get stiff in the joints and their flesh get tough when they have added birthdays to their life? Most people would answer this complex question with the remark, "because they are old." This is not the answer to why people get stiff in the joints and the flesh gets tough. The answer to premature aging is a deficiency of potassium. Over the years people never study their bodies. Nor do they learn to eat for tissue and joint youthfulness. Most peole are satisfied to eat "what agrees with them" and let it go at that . . . or they eat the foods that they were reared on and they carry these early eating habits right into their adult life.

REARING HEALTHY CHILDREN

I reared my children differently and also now my grand-children and great-grand-children are being reared by Scientific Nutrition. My children were taught how to keep themselves always in perfect physical condition so that the body tissues would continue to be soft and tender, and the elasticity of the 633 muscles and other tissues would be properly maintained. This correct way of eating would enable them to age slowly and come to the later years of life with smooth youthful-looking skin, keen hearing, sharp sparkling eyes, perfect mental and physical vitality, with absolutely no immediate signs of senility.

My children and family live in a complete state of "agelessness"! They had to learn the lessons of good nutrition. This lesson impressed the children . . . I would take an old hen and have it prepared for dinner. When the children tasted the old hen they found that the meat was tough and had a poor taste. I explained to the children that is what happens to not only poultry and beef when it is deficient in potassium, but the same thing happens to human flesh when there is a deficiency in potassium.

To prove to my children conclusively that cider vinegar and honey were an important part of their daily nutrition, I would select another old hen for the dinner table. This time in the presence of my children I would start to feed that old hen cider vinegar. I would open the hen's mouth and put two teaspoons of cider vinegar down her throat. This was done twice a day. For one week to ten days I would give the hen the vinegar ration. Then the hen was prepared for the dinner table. I would now let the children see the difference in the old hen's meat. They could see how tender it was. It was just like eating a young fowl. They found it delicious and asked for second helpings.

When the acid crystals are allowed to harden in the joints and tissues of any animal, the joints become stiff and the tissues are hardened. The meat becomes tough and tasteless. This goes for human flesh as well as animal flesh when there is a deficiency in potassium. But when apple cider vinegar programme is given them, the precipitated acid crystals enter into a solution form and pass out of the body thus making the body tissues tender.

Now when body tissues hold all the precipitated acid crystals they can, it next appears in the bursae and the joints of the body to bring on the suffering of arthritis and bursitis. For the relief of stiff aching and prematurely old joints take two teaspoons of apple cider vinegar with two teaspoons of honey in a glass of water daily. You be the judge. See how elastic and well oiled your joints will become.

26

KEEP JOINTS AND TISSUES YOUTHFUL

If you suffer from premature old joints and hardened tissues take the cider vinegar ration several times daily. this along with a balanced health diet . . . (one where 50% of the diet is composed of raw and cooked fruit and vegetables) should give tremendous benefits. Cut down on proteins, starches and sugars and see how very youthful your body will start feeling. Most people have lost their normal contact with nature and simple natural living. They no longer know how to eat the natural way.

You will find after several months of the cider vinegar and honey cocktail once or twice daily, the misery will be gone from your joints. You will discover you can walk or run up several flights of stairs without any effort. You will notice that you look younger and above all, that you feel younger than you have for years. Don't miss your potassium (cider vinegar and honey cocktail), make it a daily habit. I have seen over the years, many, many prematurely old people who were stiff in the joints with the "old age skin" transform themselves to new people. I cannot do it for you. You must make the effort to give this cider vinegar and honey programme a chance to prove what it can do for YOU!

QUESTIONS PEOPLE ASK ME ABOUT CIDER VINEGAR

Many people have some preconceived idea that pure natural apple cider vinegar is harmful to the body. Let me assure you that there is nothing in this wonderful natural product that can in anyway harm your body.

People will ask me at my Lectures when I tell of the merits and benefits of cider vinegar, they ask, "but Dr. Bragg, I've always heard that cider vinegar will thin the blood." In answering that question I always say to my alarmed students . . . "protein has a tendency to thicken the blood and the natural acids in cider vinegar help to keep the blood normal."

27

Quite naturally we find people serving **cranberry** sauce (which contains four different natural acids) along with turkey and other fowl. We find people serving apple sauce with roast pork dishes. We find people serving a slice of lemon with fish. We find people serving mushrooms with steak. The mushroom is rich in citric acid.

All these natural acids served along with protein foods are designed to lessen the thickening influence of the heavy protein. It is not a question whether the cider vinegar thins the blood or not. We should be more concerned whether the protein is thickening our blood. In order for the blood to circulate freely over the body, the blood should be thin and not thick. It is when the blood thickens that we put a strain on the heart and it is then that our blood pressure starts to go up. Remember the blood has to circulate all over the body through the arteries, blood vessels and the hair-thin capillaries. It is impossible for the blood to circulate freely through these tiny, hair-like pipes when the blood is thickened with too much protein.

Several years ago I met a woman who had extremely high blood pressure. I put her on the two day cider vinegar, honey and water programme with nothing to eat for 48 hours. She had her cider vinegar, honey and water 3 to 5 times daily. In forty-eight hours her blood pressure had dropped many points. The buzzing in the ears ceased, and her dull headache stopped. In a little over six months of correct eating (no salt, saturated fats, tea, coffee, etc.) plus her daily vinegar, honey and water programme she brought her blood-pressure down to normal.

Over the years that I have recommended the cider vinegar, honey and water programme I have had people ask me hundreds of questions about cider vinegar. They have asked me if cider vinegar dried up the blood? Would cider vinegar make me thin and skinny? I have answered these questions by saying that I have been using the cider vinegar programme for over 70 years and that it has done wonderful things to my body.

28

FOUR GENERATIONS OF HEALTHY BRAGGS –
ALL USING CIDER VINEGAR

I have fed cider vinegar to my children since they were born. My children have fed it to their children, and now my grandchildren are feeding cider vinegar to my great-grandchildren. We all use cider vinegar and unsaturated oil (peanut, soya, olive, corn, safflower oils) on our salads daily. We also use cider vinegar over cooked spinach, kale, mustard greens, chard, beet tops and many other foods.

I have recommended it to tens of thousands of my students all over the world and never once has there been reported to me one single case where cider vinegar did anything but good! So you will have nothing but good benefits from using the cider vinegar, honey and water programme.

WILL CIDER VINEGAR CURE ARTHRITIS?

First, I do not believe in cures. Curing is an internal biological function that only the body can do.

I do not offer cider vinegar as a specific for any disease or human ailment. Vinegar is part of a well-rounded programme of natural living. A scientitic natural diet, deep breathing, exercise, rest, relaxation, and all forms of natural hygiene are required to put the body in a condition to "Cure Itself." Cider vinegar is an important part of the programme. When all of the supreme forces of nature are used, the body will turn from the sick side to the well side. Health is something you must earn.

FIGHTING MUSCLE CRAMPS WITH CIDER VINEGAR

Many people are awakened in the middle of the night with sharp, painful muscle cramps. These often appear in the feet and lower or upper legs. Sometimes they appear in the stomach, intestines and sometimes in the heart. These are frightening experiences! Most people who experience cramps in the legs are forced to jump out of bed and pound the leg with the cramp up and down to get relief. Many people with cramps in other parts of the body are forced to walk fast to get relief.

When precipitated acid crystals get into the circulation of the legs and other parts of the body they cause severe cramps. I have recommended to many of these sufferers of cramps that they can get blessed relief from these painful cramps by taking two teaspoons of apple cider vinegar and two teaspoons of honey in a glass of water three times daily. This allows the precipitated acid crystals to enter into a solution form and pass out of the body, thus aiding the horrible muscle cramps to vanish.

YOU MUST FIGHT ACID CRYSTALS ALL YOUR LIFE

The healthiest person in the world must continually fight the build up of acid crystals in the body. The greatest enemy of acid crystals is the apple cider vinegar, honey, water cocktail. This powerful mixture puts the acid crystals in solution and they are flushed out of the body by the kidneys and other organs of elimination.

MAKE THIS 48 HOUR TEST

For two full days take nothing into the System but the cider vinegar and honey and water cocktail . . . use it at least three times daily during the 48 hour period, you can use it up to 5 times daily if you wish. Now after 48 hours of this programme . . . take a sample of the early morning urine you pass on the second day after you have eaten nothing for 48 hours. Put this urine sample in a bottle and put a screw top on it. Now place it on a shelf and let it stand for two weeks. Now take it out in the sunlight and examine it. You will see with your own eyes the sediment on the bottom of the bottle . . . the toxins that have been flushed out of the body!

POTASSIUM – THE MASTER MINERAL

Always keep the fact in mind that potassium puts toxic poisons in solution so they can be flushed out of the body. The body is self-healing and self-repairing. Just give it the tools to work with and you will have a painless, tireless, ageless body, regardless of your age! Forget age and calendar years . . . for age is not toxic! You age prematurely because you suffer from nutritional deficiencies and because of the fact your Vital Force is low and you have poor body drainage.

With Natural Living, you rebuild your Vital Force. Watch the transformation that will take place in your body when you are faithful with your cider vinegar, honey and water programme. You will and can create the kind of person you want to be!

All directions in this manuscript must be closely followed. Do not *try* to do everything listed here, at one time. Remember it took you a long time to cause trouble in your body by wrong habits of living. Now, it is going to take time for the body to rebuild and repair itself into a more "perfect health home" for you! Please remember after all – your body is your "home" while on this earth – so guard and protect it!!!

Many people go throughout life committing partial suicide — destroying their health, youth, beauty, talents, energies, creative qualities. Indeed, to learn how to be good to oneself is often more difficult than to learn how to be good to others.
— Paul C. Bragg

My father and I have shared the Bragg Blueprint with millions of people around the world at the Bragg Health and Fitness Crusades. I would now like to share it with those of you interested in the Apple Cigar Vinegar Health System.

With Blessings of Health, Peace & Joy,

Patricia Bragg

WE THANK THEE

For flowers that bloom about our feet;
    For song of bird and hum of bee;
For all things fair we hear or see,
    Father in heaven we thank Thee!
For blue of stream and blue of sky;
    For pleasant shade of branches high;
For fragrant air and cooling breeze;
    For beauty of the blooming trees,
Father in heaven, we thank Thee!
    For mother-love and father-care,
For brothers strong and sisters fair;
    For love at home and here each day;
For guidance lest we go astray,
    Father in heaven, we thank Thee!
For this new morning with its light;
    For rest and shelter of the night;
For health and food, for love and friends;
    For every thing His goodness sends,
Father in heaven, we thank Thee!
                    - *Ralph Waldo Emerson*

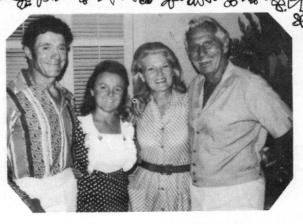

Jack LaLanne, Patricia Bragg, Elaine LaLanne & Paul Bragg

Jack says, "Bragg saved my life at age 14 when I attended the Bragg Crusades in Oakland, California." From that day on Jack has lived the health life and teaches Health & Fitness to millions.

The Bragg Blueprint for Physical, Mental & Spiritual Improvement . . . Healthy, Vital Living to 120

By

PATRICIA BRAGG, N.D., Ph.D.
LIFE EXTENSION NUTRITIONIST

Just think in 90 days you can build a new bloodstream! Not a thick, sluggish, toxic-saturated bloodstream, but a rich red bloodstream rich in all the vitamins, minerals and vital nutrients necessary for radiant and lasting health. First and foremost, we must build the Iron content of our bloodstream. As this is one of the great secrets of life the more Iron in the bloodstream, the more OXYGEN is going to flood your body, purifying everyone of the cells of your body. Oxygen is the greatest stimulant in the world. It stimulates but does not depress. All other stimulants stimulate but there is an aftermath of depression. Tobacco, alcohol, coffee, tea, refined white sugar and drugs have this effect on the body. But not God's own oxygen. So, in our Program for Self-Improvement we forever discard these above stated destroying stimulants. These are never going to enter your body! You are going to rely on the natural stimulants to create more Vital Force. First, you are going to follow the Breathing Program that is so important to this Program. You are going to use foods such as honey, fresh fruits and fresh vegetables that help build the vital blood sugar in the blood.

Before you eat or drink anything—I want you to ask yourself this important question—*"Is this going to build my bloodstream or help to destroy it?"* Be ever on the alert to protect your Stream of Life, the bloodstream! When it demands liquids, give it pure water (distilled water is the best) or live food juices such as fresh fruit and vegetable juices. Get yourself a juicer and each and every day fortify your bloodstream with fresh orange juice, grapefruit, carrot juice or a combination of different fresh juices such as celery, tomato, beet, carrot, parsley and two of the greatest juices to add with these vegetable juices—the juices of raw spinach and raw watercress. For a taste delight and a great purifier with vegetable juices, juice 1-2 garlic buds.

Do not over drink on these powerful live food juices. A pint a day is sufficient. Some people get a juicing machine and they go overboard in drinking too much juice, for overdoing your body with these juices could upset your sugar balance. Always learn to not overdo just because it is good for you—moderation in your food intake is best for building Vitality Supreme!

Just think of it—in just 11 months from now you will have an absolutely New YOU! Every one of the soft cells of the body will be renewed and there are billions of them that make hair, eyes, nose, skin, hands, feet, etc., and all the vital organs of your body. You do not need to submit to the huge risk of a heart, kidney or any other kind of transplant. You have within your power by the food you eat, the liquid you drink and by the air you breathe to build yourself a fresh vital body from the top of your head to the tip of your toes. You are what you eat and what you eat today will be walking and talking tomorrow! How wonderful our Creator has been to us, to give us the power every 90 days to build a new bloodstream and every 11 months an entirely new body. The Creator gave us the intelligence and reasoning power to control this body of ours. The Creator gave us a sharp, keen mind to think with.

FLESH IS DUMB! You can stuff almost anything in your stomach and get away with it almost! Most young people do, because youth thinks it is totally indestructible. But what a sad, sad lesson they learn as they live 40 or 50 years and the miseries and the aches and pains creep into their bodies, making their lives a living, tormenting hell on earth.

Live by the reasoning mind rather than by the senses of the body. The dumb senses are constantly enticing you to do the very things that destroy this wonderful body. Look around you—look at the horrible human sights you see! Weak people, mentally depressed people, and sickness everywhere. This pitiful condition that the average person suffers with is self-inflicted. "For whatsoever a man soweth, that shall he also reap." (Gal. 6:7) We should know and observe the fact that everything in the Universe is always governed by definite laws, with no exceptions. If we understand and follow them—we will sow the seeds of constructive healthy living!

MAKE EVERY DAY A HEALTH DAY— and each day you will improve! You will feel the new strength and energy flooding into your body. I do not have the adequate words to tell you of the feeling you will experience when you live the true natural health life. It's a feeling that is beyond description. But what a powerful and joyful feeling it is—to be fully alive, vigorous and with unlimited nerve force.

DON'T TELL ME IT'S TOO LATE FOR YOU TO BUILD RADIANT HEALTH!

Weak people find weak excuses in order to continue their bad habits of living. They will tell you they are too old to go on a Program of Self-Improvement. In the first place, I do not believe that age is a force or that it is toxic. Time is just a measure, nothing more and nothing less. We have long ago given up living in calendar years. We only live in biological years. There are plenty of people in their 30's and 40's that are biologically prematurely old. And there are plenty of people in their 60's, 70's, 80's and 90's who are biologically young.

In my opinion, if you are experiencing premature aging you are suffering from a high toxic condition and you are suffering with many nutritional deficiencies. In my opinion, that is the main cause of most human troubles. And this program will show you how to banish these two vicious enemies.

So, from this minute on, stop living by calendar years! In fact, you can just forget your birthdays as I do. All of us have birthdays every second of the day for new body cells are being born. So, away with this talk of "getting old!" From this minute on you have no age except your biological age and this you are going to control. Every day say to yourself over and over again *"I WILL NEVER GROW OLD!"* Burn it deeply in your conscious mind and above all bury it deeply into your subconscious mind.

Most people have a dreaded fear of "getting old." They picture themselves as being half-blind, with impaired hearing teeth gone, energy and vitality spent, mentally senile. They see themselves a burden to their family and friends. They see themselves in the old peoples home alone, forsaken and forgotten. People do fear old age and the train of ailments that go with "getting old." But if they only knew that they, themselves, can prevent this human tragedy. You can skip this terrible period by how you live from today on. Today is the day to prepare against senility and decrepitude. That is why I urge you to follow the wise and wonderful Laws of Mother Nature. You will grow younger as you live longer! That is what this program is all about—The Preservation of Health!

PREVENTION HELPS YOU
STAY YOUNG, VITAL AND VIRILE!

Lengthening life by special treatment of chronic miseries often means merely adding years of ill-health and misery to a person's life—what is often called "the living death." Who wants to extend life just to suffer? In my opinion, the true function of the Healer today is to prevent rather than heal. For no man is able to heal you! Only Nature can do that! In order to be healthy it is essential that everybody should know how to live in order to always be well. An ounce of prevention is worth a pound of cure!

Our greatest enemy to health is constipation! I have No Cure For Constipation! Constipation can be controlled by living on a diet that gives you plenty of bulk, moisture and lubrication and plenty of vigorous exercise of the entire abdominal cavity. In the remote parts of the world where we

36

have traveled outside the influences of so-called modern civilization, mankind indulges in the normal habit of defecation after every meal. I want you to make a habit upon arising and after each meal by training yourself to have a bowel movement. If you have children, they should be taught this habit from infancy, at home and in the schools, then constipation would be prevented.

DIET FOR HEALTH AND YOUTHFULNESS—Your diet should be composed of at least 60% raw fruit, raw vegetables and properly cooked (steamed or baked) vegetables. By this habit such conditions as stomach upsets, miseries and constipation . . . so often occuring in children and adults could be avoided! Out-go should equal intake. You should have a bowel movement upon arising and after each meal.

CONSTIPATION CREATES TOXIC POISON IN THE BODY—Studies reveal the presence of toxic poison (toxins) in cases of constipation. When these toxins are absorbed into the general circulation, the liver which is the detoxicating organ is unable to cope with them. These toxins then are thrown back in the body and cause trouble and sickness. *Toxemia is our real enemy!*

I firmly believe diet plays a very important role in the maintenance of health and the prevention of pathological conditions. I have found in my researches that diets composed of refined white flour and sugar, preserved meats such as hot dogs and lunch meats, white rice, coffee, tea, cola drinks, alcohol, margarine, over-cooked vegetables, over-cooked meats and salted foods, can bring on many miseries in the human body, especially miseries of the respiratory and the gastro-intestinal tracts. *None of these food-less foods should be eaten by You!*

WHERE YOUR ENERGY COMES FROM—The spark of life is maintained by the atomic energy contained within every single cell of the human body. It embodies electrons, protons, neutrons, positrons and alpha particles. These atoms are constantly discharging their ionic compounds as energy in work is carried out, both mental and physical, in accordance with bodily requirements. This loss of energy must be replaced. Every cell in the body is like a battery which when run down must be recharged. This is done by the intake of food and also proper breathing and exercise helps recharge the cells.

Now there are two kinds of foods, food in a low rate of physical vibration such as the foods we have mentioned—the processed, chemicalized, food-less foods such as refined white flour and sugars, etc. It is impossible to have a youthful, dynamic body when you are year after year feeding it foods and drinks with a low rate of vibration.

The Blueprint For Health Food Program will only consist of foods in a high rate of vibration. Many people have the preconceived idea that protein is the food that is in the highest rate of vibration. While protein is an important nutrient to the human body—fresh fruit is the food which has a higher rate of vibration. Fruit produces blood sugar into the blood and blood sugar is the nutrition which helps to feed the nerves of the body. Fruit has a two-fold purpose in the body. First, it is rich in blood sugar and next, it is a detoxifier of obstructions, wastes, and toxins that can do the body great harm. You will often hear people say, "I am allergic to apples, grapefruit, or peaches, or strawberries, etc.!" These people have no idea what these foods are doing in their bodies. To give you an example, my father Paul C. Bragg was reared in the South many, many years ago. His diet was rich in protein as they raised hogs, chickens, beef, sheep and fowl. Their table at each meal had a wide variety of meat proteins. Then there were hot white flour biscuits and bread, mashed and fried potatoes, and always a heavy sugary dessert. When he would eat strawberries, or tomatoes, or green peppers, or many fruits, he would break out with the most painful red itching hives. He was told he was allergic to these fruits and vegetables and therefore must avoid them. He refrained from eating these vital foods until he became a health advocate at the age of sixteen.

It was not until many years later when he perfected his Bragg Natural Method of Living that he could eat these fruits and vegetables without any reaction. Through fasting and careful nutrition he slowly detoxified himself and could eat any natural foods without fears of a violent reaction as he experienced earlier in life. As a youth his body was so saturated with toxic poisons, mucus and putrid food residues that when the cleansing-active fruits went into his body and started to cleanse—this often caused a cleansing reaction (hives, colds, headaches, aches & pains, etc.).

This is the reason everyone cannot start including a large amount of fresh fruits and raw vegetables into the diet when they have been living on a diet high in protein, starches, sugars and fats.

THE TRANSITION DIET—Everyone who wants to live the health life must thoroughly understand just what is going on in the body chemistry. First, that raw (fresh) fruit and raw (fresh) vegetables help to flush toxic poisons out of the body. But the body cannot be rushed! It takes the average person a long time to saturate the body with toxic poisons and it is going to take time for these poisons to be flushed out!

The more raw fruits and raw vegetables you have conditioned yourself to handle, the more cleansed your body will become! So, recognize raw fruit and raw vegetables as foods in the highest rate of vibration. But please respect their great cleansing action!

I often go four or five days with an abundance of my foods in mostly the raw state. Many days my schedule runs like this:

BREAKFAST: Raw fruit juice (fresh orange, grapefruit or carrot, celery, garlic, spinach, etc.) and later raw fruit (melon, apple, banana, etc.) or ... the Bragg Pep Blender Drink which is nutritious, delicious and easy and fast to prepare: 1 glass juice (orange, pineapple, apple, etc.), 1-2 ripe bananas or fruit in season, 1 tbsp Brewer's yeast, 1 tsp Lecithin granules, 1 tbsp Protein Soy Powder, ½ tsp Vitamin C powder, 1 tsp raw sunflower seeds, ½ tsp raisins. Blend—if you want chilled, add ice cube in blender. You can vary this drink to your desires and needs.

LUNCH: Large raw combination vegetable, sprouts and green salad, a few raw nuts or seeds.

DINNER: Salad first—then two steamed or baked fresh vegetables and one of the following: beans, lentils, brown rice, whole grain pasta, baked or steamed potato.

Remember to get your daily Apple Cider Vinegar into your diet: Apple Cider Vinegar Cocktail; over salad, steamed greens, etc.

Now, you know what people are told today—first, that they must start the day with a big breakfast as this will give great energy in the morning hours where energy is needed badly. So, they gorge themselves on a big breakfast mostly consisting of a big bowl of processed cereal with cream and sugar, ham and eggs, or bacon and eggs, hot cakes, stacks of buttered toast, jam, jelly, and all this washed down with coffee, milk, or cocoa. You will note there is no fruit at this meal. It is a concentration of starch, protein and fat. It will take the digestive system hours to work on this mass of concentrated processed food. All the vital energy of the body will be needed for this great task of digestion. So, I ask you "How in the name of common sense can a big meal like this give a person strength for the morning duties?" The truth of the matter is it can't. This is how the housewives and mothers are brain-washed by the big food interests who have all this food-less food to sell.

Only a person doing the most strenuous physical labor could possible burn a meal like this up. And even I have my doubts. Now you know why there is so much indigestion and constipation. These heavy fat, starch, protein and sugar breakfasts lay on the stomach like a ton of bricks, and then they have to dynamite it out. Laxatives are one of the biggest sellers in drug stores.

YOU MUST CHANGE YOUR IDEAS ABOUT FOOD. It is not a matter of how much you eat but the kind of food you eat. Make it a point to eat smaller amounts of food, but—eat an abundance of those foods with a high rate of vibration.

FASTING—THE MASTER KEY TO INTERNAL PURIFICATION

If you will take a complete water fast for 24 hours each week, soon you will find you can add more fresh fruit and vegetables to your diet. And after a fast of 3 to 7 days you can even include more of the foods that are in a high rate of vibration.

I faithfully fast for 24 hours each week and then I also do longer fasts from 3, 7 and 10 days and wait 'til you experience this—you will love the pure feeling you receive!

FASTING BRINGS REMARKABLE RESULTS — from animals to even worms—states Professor A.E. Crews of Edinburgh University. "Given appropriate and essential conditions of the environment, including proper care of the body, and Eternal Youth is in fact a reality in living forms. It's found to be possible by repeated processes of fasting, to keep a worm alive twenty times longer than it would have lived in the regular way. This has also been proven with animals." This gives you something to think about.

Remember it took time for the body to build up the toxins—so it takes time to unload them—to take your time—and be faithful to your Health Program, it will bring many wonderful benefits. Cut down on all concentrated foods gradually. If you eat meat—*do not eat meat more than three times a week.* Meat has uric acid, urea, and saturated fats. These are all highly toxic materials and are not good for the body. Substitute fish some days as it is a cleaner protein than meat and a less saturated fat, and also chicken and turkey which have far less uric acid, urea and saturated fat than meat.

There are many other good proteins in the vegetable kingdom. The soy bean is an excellent protein, also brown and wild rice. So are all the many varieties of beans, such as dried lima beans, garbanzos, split peas, lentils, pinto beans, kidney beans, etc. Remember that beans are a good source of magnesium which is so necessary to your heart and good nutritional health.

Eggs should not be eaten over 4 times weekly. They are a highly concentrated food with a saturated fat (cholesterol builder) in the yolk, and if a person has a high cholesterol count (over 225) it's best to leave eggs out of your diet completely. The same goes for cheeses, as they are highly concentrated, and if eaten—be sure it is the naturally aged cheese and not the processed cheese, and even then should only be eaten sparingly. If you are prone to a mucus condition then all milk products and eggs are best left out of your diet!

If you have been used to eating an unbalanced breakfast, start to include more fresh fruit and *slowly cut down* on the concentrated foods. If you have been used to eating bacon or ham and white flour breads, sweet rolls, etc.—now leave these processed and preserved foods as they are foods with an extremely low rate of vibration. Instead of eating two eggs per day, eat only one and soon you can cut down to only four per week.

Stewed prunes and raw wheat germ and honey with fresh fruit make a good, nutritious breakfast. But in time you should learn to live on a no-breakfast plan. Generally, you do not need this food. There were no two people any more active physically and mentally than my father and I, and we never ate breakfast—unless you want to call fresh fruit a breakfast. But before we even ate fresh fruit we did all our morning exercises, our deep breathing, or had a long hike or swim. Our day usually began around 5 a.m. and we were busy until 10 a.m. or later before we even ate our fresh fruit. Many mornings we were so busy with some mental and physical activity that we did not even take the time to eat our fresh fruit.

I believe most people over-eat! And that is the reason their vitality is at such a low ebb. So—do not over-do on eating—even if it is good health foods. Just remember a toxic body requires a large amount of food. When they eat, the body is forced to work on the digestion of this food and has no energy for detoxification. So the toxins pile up and they accumulate their physical miseries and their premature aging. These toxins are obstructions and are the mischief makers.

THE "SECRET" OF HEALTH
LIES IN INTERNAL CLEANLINESS

That is what you want to strive for—a toxicless body! So, gradually include more fresh fruit and raw vegetables into your diet. Have your fresh fruit in the morning and your raw combination vegetable salad at noon with fresh fruit for dessert if desired. Eat a cooked yellow vegetable every day such as yam, sweet potato, yellow squash of all kinds or cooked carrots. Then a steamed or baked green vegetable. Then with your main meal you may have some kind of protein such as meat, fish, eggs, natural cheese or the vegetarian proteins such as soy beans, nuts, etc., sunflowers and sesame seeds and avocados, etc. Have beans at least once a week. By having a variety of the natural foods, this is the best way to enjoy a balanced menu.

You may use the natural oils such as olive, soy bean, safflower, peanut, corn or sesame. Be sure the oils are not preserved. Read the label carefully before buying. I like to put olive oil over my baked potato, instead of butter. Also a little oil over your baked beans is delicious—with a sprinkle of kelp seasoning and parmesan cheese. I do not use salt. The best way to eat potatoes is baked. I use the fast method of baking. Thoroughly scrub the potato (either white, yam or sweet) and do not wrap or oil. Bake it in a hot oven 450 degrees for 25 minutes. This converts the starch of the potato to a blood sugar. The skin must be eaten also . . . it's delicious and so crunchy baked this fast way.

Salt has no place in your diet! Salt is an inorganic substance and only causes mischief in the body. Read labels and if products contain salt, do not buy them!

AVOID FOOD-LESS, PROCESSED FOODS!

Eliminate refined white flour products and white sugar products entirely. No mushy, dead, refined cereals or those dry commercial cereals—for they are in a low rate of vibration, regardless how they have been enriched with chemical vitamins and minerals. (Health Stores carry natural organic cereals if you desire a hot natural-grain cereal.)

Avoid all these: • Fried foods • Frozen foods
• Salted foods • Refined, preserved, chemicalized foods
• Coffee, tea, cola drinks, alcohol, or sugared, salted juices
• Over-cooked, over-salted vegetables, and salted creamed flour-thickened soups.

You now know the foods you can eat (fresh fruits, fresh juices, salads, fresh vegetables steamed or baked and if you eat meat—not over three times a week, other days fish, fowl or vegetable proteins.)

You now know the foods you cannot eat (food-less, processed, chemicalized foods and beverages.)

Use your imagination to plan live-food meals which are in a high rate of vibration. Above all, eat simply and occasionally go a full day on only fruits. Avoid too many mixtures; do not over-eat; be moderate in all things for the best of health. And only eat when you are really hungry, not because it is meal-time. Earn your food by activity and vigorous exercise and deep breathing. You will see how much more you enjoy your meal-time when you earn your food by activity.

THE POWERFUL SOURCE OF FRUIT. Always keep in mind the most perfect food for man is fresh, ripe fruit. Nature in her inimitable way, brings together in her fruits, a marvelously-balanced, living combination of vital principles, in a high rate of vibration, bio-magnetized, to release the living building blocks so necessary for live body function. Tinted by the basking rays of the vitalizing sun, breathing in draughts of magnetized air, drawing to itself the vital minerals dug out of the earth by the roots of its bearer, fruit stands out supreme as the master stroke of perfection in the electro-chemical laboratory of Nature, whom we had best call God! Man can take all the chemicals of an apple out of a chemist's dish, but he cannot construct an apple! He may analyze all the minerals of a cherry, but he doesn't even know what makes them red. He may take apart and try to reconstruct a grape, and find that the grape supports life and the broken-down chemicals do not! Fruit contains certain bio-electric principles that give the electric spark of life which no other food prepared by Nature possesses quite as perfectly. Fruit is the most perfect food of Nature, and will support life indefinitely to a superior degree, when a body is entirely cleansed and living in a completely natural environment.

Who has not had his "mouth water" when seeing a luscious dish of fruit before him—for instance a couple of yellow pears with a dash of pink, or a beautiful bunch of tapering grapes, green or red or blue? The sight of fruit and the taste more so, bring an abundant secretion of digestive juices, for they are natural foods of man. Fruit is, without reserve, designed particularly well for the digestive tract of man.

I have seen a sick person turn all other food down and drink a glass of freshly squeezed orange juice. This is what his sick body craved. The vital nutrients which are found in a ripe, juicy orange. I have seen children torn with fever ask for a glass of orange juice. Why didn't they ask for a hot dog sandwich?

On the whole, a diet of only fruits as a continuous diet, is impractical and inefficient for the average American. It would be splendid in a tropical climate. But man has come so far from his perfect state that he cannot maintain an efficient standard as a fruitarian.

EAT MORE FRESH FRUIT. As I have stated, fruit makes an ideal breakfast. Honey may be added when fruit is not sweet enough as in the case with so much fruit which has not been tree ripened. Along with fresh fruit in the fall, winter and spring, eat organically grown dates, sun-dried figs, raisins and apricots.

*THE MIRACLE FOOD—"THE AVOCADO"—*stands high as a miracle food of nature. First, the avocado tree is strong and insects do not bother it. It requires no spraying with poisonous chemicals. The avocado has a perfect balance of life-giving nutrients. It has an unsaturated fat which the body can handle perfectly. I use avocados practically every day of my life when I can get them. I wait until they ripen and then cut in half, seed and peel them, and I like to mash them up and then I take my garlic press and squeeze fresh garlic over the mashed avocado. With sliced tomatoes, celery, carrot sticks, lettuce leaves, radish, cucumber, green bellpepper, this makes a delicious high vibration lunch meal.

I use ripe bananas in my diet. It is not a fattening fruit as supposed. It consists of 70% water. Apples of all kinds make excellent eating, as do pears and grapes. Eat fruit and see how wonderful you will feel and look!

FOODS IN A HIGH VIBRATION
CONTAIN LIFE-GIVING SUBSTANCE

When you eat only foods which are in a high vibration your body performs and operates under God's Universal Law and becomes ● Self-starting ● Self-governing ● Self-generating instrument! I want you to live under the Universal Laws of Nature so your body will be a fine working instrument. To YOU, young or old, who desire to retain the vivacity, vitality, energy and enthusiasm of youth and who desire to turn back the clock of Father Time, whose bodies are bent, whose eyes are dimmed, who walk with a halting gait at an age when you should be buoyant with the spirit of youth *there is but one way to live and that is NATURE'S WAY!*

Old age is just a highly toxic condition—plus nutritional deficiencies. Premature death is often an unnecessary tragedy.
- This is an Age of AGELESSNESS. You can be a part of it!
- The Spirit of Youth is now a vital necessity everywhere! Old men and women are not wanted. Many times they are in the way. They are sometimes an encumbrance to themselves and everyone with whom they come in contact. Years may have crept up upon you. You may have advanced far into what is considered old age. But do not despair. You may regain not only the spirit, but much of the vigor of youth, and it is your duty to do so!

Square your shoulders and look life squarely in the face. Keep premature aging out of your body by following a Program of Natural Living which means eating foods having a high rate of vibration (abundance of raw fruits and vegetables), deep breathing, exercise, and one day a week of water fasting, 8 hours of restful sleep at night and keep the body relaxed, don't let anything rob you of your emotional and nervous energy.

Your body is being made over every day, and premature aging and senility results from the debris that accumulates in the process of rebuilding. Maintain proper activity of your body throughout every part, and there will be little or no debris.

Act the part of youth. Cultivate and rigidly hold on to the Spirit of Youth! Maintain your energies at high-level mark. Keep your spine straight. Thus premature aging will find no opportunity to enter your life. If you are already in the clutches of premature aging, begin now to fight for the return of youth. Work with might and main for restoration of this priceless possession. Train your body as you would that of a race horse. Follow out the clear and definite instructions that will give you strength, virility, energy, vivacity, enthusiasm, and make your life a daily enjoyment for the most precious of all earthly gifts—the power, and joys of youthful, healthful living. Men and women have been young at 50, 60, 70, 80, and even 90. Some have retained the Spirit of Youth beyond the century mark. Those who live in accordance with God's Universal Laws maintain that life grows more beautiful year by year; that its glories, its joys, its delights increase with age.

If you are living the incomplete life, if you are giving up the precious things of human existence for the drunken stupor of dietetic excesses, for the pleasures of luxury, idleness of ease, you are selling your birthright for a mess of potage.

Wake up to the possibilities within your reach! Rejuvenate your body. Make your mind keen and capable. Obey the Laws of Nature and you will achieve results that you now scarcely dare to dream.

SUGGESTIONS FOR A DAILY PROGRAM

Be sure to thoroughly ventilate your sleeping room so you will get a large amount of oxygen while sleeping. Be sure you sleep in a spread-out position to allow for good circulation. Do not sleep in a cramped position or sleep on your arm or shoulder, spread out completely. Your mattress should be firm and flat.

Oxygen is the life of the blood, and the blood is the life of the body. A person weighing about 150 pounds, contains about 88 pounds of oxygen. Oxygen is the most important chemical of the body. Yet it is colorless, odorless, and tasteless. Its main function is purification. Lack of oxygen in the body can lead to serious consequences and the majority of people are oxygen-starved for they are shallow breathers.

To have a Youthful, Vital Life we need air in abundance, pure distilled water, and plenty of fresh vegetables and fruits. Oxygen is an unquestionable source of indispensable energy necessary for higher vital activity in the human organism. It insures elimination, reconstruction and regeneration within the vital factors and the metabolic activities of the physical body.

Through the function of the lungs, the oxygen is absorbed, transformed and assimilated into the blood, bringing with it unknown factors in the vital forces of the atmosphere.

I know that plant life through its roots in the ground absorbs all the vital elements in the soil necessary for the life of plants and that if I cut or interfere with their roots—they die! Man's roots are his lungs.

There can be no adequate breathing without much physical movement. Without the proper physical movements one cannot be physically motivated to obtain the full elixir of life which is the breath of air. The stronger and more virile our movements are, the more air we need and the greater is our rate of breath acceleration. The oxygen in the air that we breath dissolves and eliminates waste and builds the continum of our cellular structure, thus maintaining our organism to the highest degree possible. Each breath should detoxify and regenerate our vital forces. This must be completely supplemented, however, by the correct natural foods that I advocate.

I want it definitely understood neither exercise nor conscious deep breathing can prevent the process of degeneration of the cells unless proper nutrition is added for fortification.

This explains why even some of the top athletes who do not follow a correct nutritional balanced diet decline in their late twenties and thirties. There are maybe a few exceptions but the average athlete reaches his peak at about 27 and then the decline begins. I know this to be true, as my father was an active athlete for over 75 years and we saw the finest athletes reach their peak and then slowly decline with many dying young.

Other Factors Affecting BREATHING—thoughts and emotions interfere with our breathing. That is why, should we have a headache, or other suddenly-arising symptoms, by a few minutes of deep conscious breathing exercises in the open air will speedily help detoxify and re-establish balance for the time being and help relieve ourselves of our miseries.

Upon waking in the morning, stretch the legs and arms and body as you do when yawning. Continue this stretching process until you feel that every muscle has been properly and thoroughly awakened. Good circulation is the master key to good health! That is the reason it is important to stretch and exercise your body. And don't do exercises just in the morning, take some time during the day—to keep your circulation whirling during your waking hours. Keep that blood whirling at top speed throughout the pipes of the body. Do not sit longer than one hour at a time. Get up and move around. *To rest is to rust and rust is destruction!* Don't sit in a car for more than an hour—stop the car and get out and stretch and exercise your legs and body.

EXERCISES HELP KEEP YOU YOUTHFUL, FLEXIBLE AND TRIM

It is stiffness which we must fight off, if you want the body to feel young. To a large extent, the prematurely old man and woman finds it impossible to straighten their spine or hold a good posture continually for they become stiff and rigid through lack of exercise and use.

It is no wonder that men and women become prematurely old, and settle down, and get crusty and "stiff-necked" (literally). They do not do exercises that move their spinal joints! If you have already begun to acquire this condition of stiffness, take warning right now! Right about face! *GO TO WORK ON YOURSELF* and strive for flexibility and elasticity in every part of your body, especially your spine! Now, you have a real job for yourself—to develop a flexible and elastic spine. Your figure can look ten years younger if you will keep your spine active. Youthful looking people have good postures. The key to posture improvements is attention to the spine. The spine is a marvelous "instrument" and is the central support of the whole body. It is made up of a flexible column of squarish bones which are joined together with rubbery puffs called discs. This wonderful piece of human equipment stores its own lubrication in little sacs at the joints. The spine was designed for action! By keeping it loose and supple, our whole body moves with grace, ease and youthfulness.

"I have found a perfect health, a new state of existence, a feeling of purity and happiness, something unknown to humans . . ."

—Novelist Upton Sinclair,
who fasted frequently.

YOUR WAIST-LINE IS YOUR LIFE-LINE
AND YOUR DATE-LINE!

Today I want you to get a tape measure and measure your waist. Write your waist measurement down and check it daily and in short time you will see a more trim and youthful waist-line through vigorous exercise of the abdomen area. And of course correct eating and your 24-hour weekly fast and later on longer 3, 5 or 7 day fasts. This will surely help your waist-line, along with exercise and correct diet. *A slender, trim waist-line makes a person appear years younger* — so let's get yours down to where it should be — if it has grown too big and fat. It is a trim horse for the long race they say — and I am sure we all want to be here for a long time! Living this health life is so wonderful — truly, life is beautiful!

People abuse their abdomens abominably! You cannot eat dead-empty-calorie foods and tell yourself that a tiny snack here, and there won't show! You are wrong. Dead-devitalized foods create toxic poisons inside your body and this all helps to add flabby inches to the abdomen. Do not over-eat even the correct foods—your body only needs enough food to maintain energy—and when you stuff too much fuel into it—then you see fat people walking around—you know they are not burning up the excess.

You are not getting away with this kind of cheating—it's just cheating (hurting) yourself! Bear in mind as we live longer, the internal abdominal structure and stomach muscles relax more. This is called visceroptosis, or droopy tummy, and it is a common ailment among older people who do not exercise those waist muscles. It can be a contributing cause of constipation, sluggish liver and even hernias.

When the abdominal wall becomes lazy and the consequent droop is compounded by a few layers of flab, trouble starts on the inside of the abdomen. Most people by the time they have reached 40 have a complete prolapsed abdomen. Start looking at people and you will notice what I am saying—is the truth!

So, don't let your abdomen drop, make every effort to bring it back to firmness again. . . . it responds quickly to exercises.

MAINTAIN THE POSTURE OF YOUTH

There is a fundamental relationship between good posture and youth on the one hand, and bent posture and age, on the other. To maintain the posture of youth actually means the maintenance of youth itself, because of the basic relationship between the healthy normal spine and the condition of bodily vigor which signifies youth, irrespective of how many years one has lived.

As has been already noted, the most easily recognized sign of premature aging is the forward bend of the spine, combined with the "round shoulders" which necessarily accompany it. Prematurely old people often exhibit this condition in a very marked degree, almost bending over double. But people sometimes show this sign of premature aging rather early in life. On the other hand, people of advanced years, by simply straightening their spines and walking erect, make themselves look ten to thirty years younger than they really are. Look around you and start noticing postures and you will see what we mean!

Therefore, it may be said, one's entire life should be a constant fight to maintain correct erect position. Remember that the spine is the fundamental structure of the human body. With the brain, in which it starts, it constitutes the center of the nervous system. All other parts of the body are, so to speak, appendages of the spine. The shoulders and arms at the upper end, and the hips and legs at the other, are simply tacked onto the spine. If you did not have a spine, you would be a jellyfish, a shellfish, or an insect. Keep that spinal column straight, keep it flexible and keep it erect! Good health and longevity depends on an erect body. Go to your full length mirror and take a good look at your posture and then start working on it!

GOOD POSTURE CHECK—Stand against the wall with heels, buttocks, waist (draw in waist and push back against wall), and shoulders and head touching the wall—then walk away from the wall, holding this straight position. Do this several times during the day and try and hold this posture as long as possible. Soon you will retrain your muscles to stand straight.

STOP DYING — START LIVING

The Bible tells us that *"THE KINGDOM OF HEAVEN IS WITHIN,"* and this statement I thoroughly believe. We can either make this body we live in a kingdom of heaven or we can make it a torture chamber.

What kind of body you will live in is strictly up to you! I cannot live your life for you. Nor can anyone else! You are a mature adult, and you must face the reality of life. You have the will power and desire, I am sure, to follow this program— so do, start today!

This is a Master Blueprint to Physical Perfection because it works with the Laws of God and Nature. God and Nature make no compromises. You either follow the good laws of God and Nature or you try and break them! You cannot break a natural law or a God law — for it only breaks you in your foolish attempt.

FOLLOW THESE NATURAL LAWS
FOR PHYSICAL PERFECTION

These Laws God put in motion are perfect Laws created for your own good:
- You must eat Natural Foods
- You must breath deeply of God's air.
- You must exercise the 640 muscles of your body.
- You must give it pure clean water.
- You must give your body sunshine (sunbaths).
- You must not over-work your body as this leads to stress, strains and tensions and nerve depletion.
- You must keep the body clean outside and inside.
- You must live by intelligence and wisdom.

We are creatures of a Perfect Creator. As such there must be inherent in us the potentiality to become physically perfect. It must be the intent of our Perfect Creator to have us physically perfect!

If it is the will of our Perfect Creator that we be physically perfect, then when we are not physically perfect we are out of harmony with the creative design, and therefore, out of harmony with God's intent, will or law. In other and simpler words, we are, in our living habits, opposing the will of God.

So, you see that to reach physical perfection we must live on all three planes: *THE PHYSICAL, THE MENTAL AND THE SPIRITUAL.* By living on the physical plane correctly we automatically reach a higher state of mentality and spirituality.

If you eat God and Nature's natural foods and build a rich red clean bloodstream you are going to be keener mentally. And the wonderful part of living by God and Nature's Blueprint—is we find a new calmness coming over us. You find you experience a new feeling of confidence, of peace and serenity. When every cell, organ and body part are functioning perfectly, the body must be perfect, physically, mentally and spiritually. What complete satisfaction you will feel when you are living this health life and reaping the great rewards!

Your degree of physical perfection is the measure of your efforts in cooperating (by daily proper diet, exercise, deep breathing and youthful thinking) with your Creator's design or intent, that you become and remain physically perfect regardless of your age.

THE BODY MUST OBEY YOUR MIND

Flesh is dumb! You can put anything in your stomach from pickles to hot dogs. It is not the stomach that rules the body it is an intelligence and reasoning mind. Let me close this Blueprint with the unequivocal statement that the properly directed mind can make the body follow this program, therefore it can help in making the body physically perfect. *That is our goal — PHYSICAL PERFECTION!*

Yours for Physical Perfection, Vitality Supreme and Long-Lasting Youthfulness,

Patricia Bragg

"Open thou mine eyes, that I may behold wondrous things out of thy law."

—Psalms 119:18

53

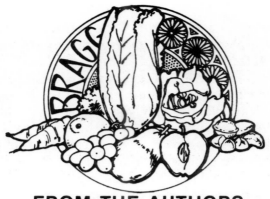

FROM THE AUTHORS

This book was written for YOU. It can be your passport to the Good Life. We Professional Nutritionists join hands in one common objective — a high standard of health for all and many added years to your life. Scientific Nutrition points the way — Nature's Way — the only lasting way to build a body free of degenerative diseases and premature aging. This book teaches you how to work with Nature and not against her. Doctors, dentists, and others who care for the sick, try to repair depleted tissues which too often mend poorly if at all. Many of them praise the spreading of this new scientific message of natural foods and methods for long-lasting health and youthfulness at any age. To speed the spreading of this tremendous message, this book was written.

Statements in this book are recitals of scientific findings, known facts of physiology, biological therapeutics, and reference to ancient writings as they are found. Paul C. Bragg has been practicing the natural methods of living for over 70 years, with highly beneficial results, knowing they are safe and of great value to others, and his daughter Patricia Bragg works with him to carry on the Health Crusade. They make no claims as to what the methods cited in this book will do for one in any given situation, and assume no obligation because of opinions expressed.

No cure for disease is offered in this book. No foods or diets are offered for the treatment or cure of any specific ailment. Nor is it intended as, or to be used as, literature for any food product. Paul C. Bragg and Patricia Bragg express their opinions solely as Public Health Educators, Professional Nutritionists and Teachers.

Certain persons considered experts may disagree with one or more statements in this book, as the same relate to various nutritional recommendations. However, any such statements are considered, nevertheless, to be factual, as based upon long-time experience of Paul C. Bragg and Patricia Bragg in the field of human health.

SEND FOR IMPORTANT
FREE HEALTH BULLETINS

Patricia Bragg, from time to time sends News Bulletins on latest Health and Nutrition Discoveries. These are sent *free of charge!*

If you wish to receive these *free bulletins* and The Health Builder—please send your name and also names of any friends and relatives you wish.

HEALTH SCIENCE Box 7, Santa Barbara, California 93102 U.S.A.

Name

Address

City   State   Zip Code

Name

Address

City   State   Zip Code

Name

Address

City   State   Zip Code

Name

Address

City   State   Zip Code

Name

Address

City   State   Zip Code

PLEASE CUT ALONG DOTTED LINE

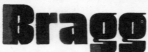

HEALTH SCIENCE
ISBN Prefix 0-87790

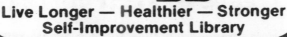

Live Longer — Healthier — Stronger
Self-Improvement Library

Let Legendary PAUL C. BRAGG, World Health Crusader, Pioneer Nutritionist, Originator of Health Stores and Beloved Sage to Millions and PATRICIA BRAGG, Health and Fitness Educator, Show You the Simple Path to a Greater, Longer, More Vital Life—"High Health" Physically, Mentally and Spiritually!

BRAGG "HOW-TO, SELF-HEALTH" BOOKS

—— Vegetarian Gourmet Health Recipes (no salt, no sugar) .... $ 4.95
—— Bragg's Complete Health Gourmet Recipes—448 pages 6.95
—— The Miracle of Fasting (Bragg Bible of Health).................................. 6.95
—— Complete Triathlon Endurance Training Manual—600 pgs .... Soft cover 16.95
     (This Bragg Health/Fitness Encyclopedia is a must reading for all!)
___ Building Powerful Nerve Force 4.95
___ How to Keep the Heart Healthy and Fit at Any Age 4.95
___ The Golden Keys to Internal Physical Fitness 2.95
___ The Natural Way to Reduce 4.95
___ The Shocking Truth About Water 4.95
___ Your Health and Your Hair 4.95
___ Healthful Eating Without Confusion 4.95
___ Salt-Free Sauerkraut Recipes 2.95
___ Nature's Healing System to Improve Eyesight in 90 days 4.95
___ Building Strong Feet... 4.95
___ Super Brain Breathing for Vital Living 3.95
___ Toxicless Diet—Purification & Healing System (Stay Ageless Program)......... 3.95
___ Powerful Health Uses of Apple Cider Vinegar 3.95
___ Building Health & Youthfulness 1.75
___ Natural Method of Physical Culture 1.75
___ Nature's Way to Health—Live 100 Active Years 1.75
___ Fitness/Spine Motion Program—Flexible, Painfree Back 1.95
___ The Philosophy of Super Health 1.75
___ South Sea Abdomen Culture for Perfect Elimination & Trim Waist 1.75

TOTAL NO.   TOTAL AMT.
—— COPIES   Prices subject to change without notice. ENCLOSED $_____

BRAGG LIQUID AMINOS—Nutrition you need . . . taste you will love . . . a family favorite for 65 years. A source of delicious, nutritious life-renewing protein. Add to casseroles, soups, sauces, gravies, potatoes, popcorn, and vegetables. An ideal "pick-me-up" broth at work, home or the gym. Tastes better than Soy & Tamari sauce. Start today and add more Amino Acids for healthy living to your daily diet—the easy BRAGG LIQUID AMINOS Way!

SIZE	PRICE	POSTAGE & HANDLING	CASE (12 Bottles) Free Freight
16 oz.	$3.95	$2.25 (UPS)	$47.04
32 oz.	$6.45	$2.75 (UPS)	$77.40

Available at most good Health Stores or from Health Science

Remember . . . The Gift of a Bragg Book is A Gift of Life!

Buy these Bragg Books today for yourself, family, and friends. Purchase or order at your Health Store, Christian Book Store or better Book Store. If unavailable in your area, order direct from Health Science. For book mail orders, please add $1.25 for first book, and 50¢ for each additional book. Add $2.00 for Triathlon book. Please add postage for Aminos as listed above. Book orders over $25 are postage free. Remittance in U.S. funds only... or use Mastercard or Visa. For Phone Orders (Visa/MC only): (805) 968-1020. California residents please add sales tax.

HEALTH SCIENCE
Box 7, Santa Barbara, California 93102 U.S.A. ⟨3 John: 2⟩

BPR-

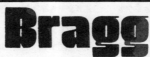

HEALTH SCIENCE
ISBN Prefix 0-87790

Bragg

Live Longer — Healthier — Stronger
Self-Improvement Library

Let Legendary PAUL C. BRAGG, World Health Crusader, Pioneer Nutritionist, Originator of Health Stores and Beloved Sage to Millions and PATRICIA BRAGG, Health and Fitness Educator, Show You the Simple Path to a Greater, Longer, More Vital Life—"High Health" Physically, Mentally and Spiritually!

BRAGG "HOW-TO, SELF-HEALTH" BOOKS

____ Vegetarian Gourmet Health Recipes (no salt, no sugar) ....$ 4.95
____ Bragg's Complete Health Gourmet Recipes—448 pages 6.95
____ The Miracle of Fasting (Bragg Bible of Health) 6.95
____ Complete Triathlon Endurance Training Manual—600 pgs...................Soft cover 16.95
       (This Bragg Health/Fitness Encyclopedia is a must reading for all!)
____ Building Powerful Nerve Force...............................4.95
____ How to Keep the Heart Healthy and Fit at Any Age 4.95
____ The Golden Keys to Internal Physical Fitness 2.95
____ The Natural Way to Reduce 4.95
____ The Shocking Truth About Water 4.95
____ Your Health and Your Hair 4.95
____ Healthful Eating Without Confusion 4.95
____ Salt-Free Sauerkraut Recipes 2.95
____ Nature's Healing System to Improve Eyesight in 90 days 4.95
____ Building Strong Feet...............................4.95
____ Super Brain Breathing for Vital Living 3.95
____ Toxicless Diet—Purification & Healing System (Stay Ageless Program)...............................3.95
____ Powerful Health Uses of Apple Cider Vinegar 3.95
____ Building Health & Youthfulness 1.75
____ Natural Method of Physical Culture 1.75
____ Nature's Way to Health—Live 100 Active Years 1.75
____ Fitness/Spine Motion Program—Flexible, Painfree Back 1.95
____ The Philosophy of Super Health 1.75
____ South Sea Abdomen Culture for Perfect Elimination & Trim Waist 1.75

____ TOTAL NO.   TOTAL AMT.
       COPIES   Prices subject to change without notice.   ENCLOSED $_____

BRAGG LIQUID AMINOS—Nutrition you need . . . taste you will love . . . a family favorite for 65 years. A source of delicious, nutritious life-renewing protein. Add to casseroles, soups, sauces, gravies, potatoes, popcorn, and vegetables. An ideal "pick-me-up" broth at work, home or the gym. Tastes better than Soy & Tamari sauce. Start today and add more Amino Acids for healthy living to your daily diet—the easy BRAGG LIQUID AMINOS Way!

SIZE	PRICE	POSTAGE & HANDLING	CASE (12 Bottles) Free Freight
16 oz.	$3.95	$2.25 (UPS)	$47.04
32 oz.	$6.45	$2.75 (UPS)	$77.40

Available at most good Health Stores or from Health Science

Remember . . . The Gift of a Bragg Book is A Gift of Life!

Buy these Bragg Books today for yourself, family, and friends. Purchase or order at your Health Store, Christian Book Store or better Book Store. If unavailable in your area, order direct from Health Science. For book mail orders, please add $1.25 for first book, and 50¢ for each additional book. Add $2.00 for Triathlon book. Please add postage for Aminos as listed above. Book orders over $25 are postage free. Remittance in U.S. funds only... or use Mastercard or Visa. For Phone Orders (Visa/MC only): (805) 968-1020. California residents please add sales tax.

HEALTH SCIENCE
Box 7, Santa Barbara, California 93102 U.S.A.

BPR-

PATRICIA BRAGG, N.D., Ph.D.

Lecturer and Author
Nutritionist, Educator, Health & Fitness Consultant
Advisor to World Leaders, Glamorous Hollywood Stars,
Singers, Dancers and Athletes

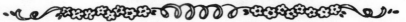

Daughter of the world renowned health authority, Paul C. Bragg, Patricia Bragg has won international fame on her own in this field. She conducts Health and Fitness Seminars for women's, men's, youth and church groups throughout the United States . . . and is co-lecturer with Paul C. Bragg on tours throughout the English speaking world. Consultants to Presidents and Royalty, to Stars of Stage, Screen and TV, and to Champion Athletes, Patricia Bragg and her father are authors and co-authors of the Bragg Health Library of instructive, inspiring books.

Patricia Bragg herself is the symbol of perpetual youth, a living and sparkling example of hers and her father's precepts.

A fifth generation Californian on her mother's side, Patricia Bragg was reared by the Natural Health Method from infancy. In school, she not only excelled in athletics but also won high honors in her studies and her counseling. She is an accomplished musician and dancer . . . as well as tennis player, swimmer and mountain climber . . . and the youngest woman ever to be granted a U.S. Patent. Patricia Bragg is a popular gifted Health Teacher and a dynamic, in-demand Talk Show Guest. In the past few years she has been featured on over 300 radio talk shows spreading simple easy-to-follow health teachings for everyone. Man's body is the Temple of the Holy Spirit, and our Creator wants us filled with Joy and Health for a long walk with him for Eternity. The Bragg Crusade of Health and Fitness (3 John 2) has carried her around the world . . . spreading health and joy physically, spiritually and mentally. Health is our birthright, and Patricia teaches how to prevent the destruction of our health from man-made wrong habits of living.

She has been Health Consultant to that great walker, President Harry S. Truman, and to the British Royal Family. Betty Cuthbert, Australia's "Golden Girl" who holds 16 world records and four Olympic gold medals in women's track, follows Patricia Bragg's guidance. Among those who come to her for advice are some of Hollywood's top stars from Clint Eastwood and family to the singing stars of the Metropolitan Opera. Patricia's message is of world-wide appeal to people of all ages, nationalities and walks-of-life who read her books and attend her Crusades.

Jesus said: "Thy faith hath made thee whole, and go and sin no more." And that means your dietetic sins. He himself, through fasting and prayer, was able to heal the sick and cure all manner of diseases.

Dear friend, I wish above all things that thou may prosper and be in health even as the soul prosper—
3 John 2